Change Your Nutrition, Change Your Life

How to Change Your Nutrition Habits for Good: A Quick Self-Help Guide

Matthew Baltzer

complete information. No warranties of any kind are declared or implied. Readers acknowledge that the author is not engaged in the rendering of legal, financial, medical or professional advice. The content within this book has been derived from various sources. Please consult a licensed professional before attempting any techniques outlined in this book.

By reading this document, the reader agrees that under no circumstances is the author responsible for any losses, direct or indirect, that are incurred as a result of the use of the information contained within this document, including, but not limited to, errors, omissions, or inaccuracies.

Table of Contents

Introduction

When it comes to dieting, most of us either know someone who has tried going on a 'diet' or have experienced trying out one or two of them ourselves. We are probably all familiar with the "Atkins Diet," the "South Beach Diet," or the "Paleo Diet." These diets all have some health benefits, and positive results are usually experienced, particularly when in the first stages of the program. However, it is probably safe to say that the majority of people who begin diets such as these more often than not 'abandon ship!' within a few weeks, or even days, of beginning. Why is this something that happens so often? The truth of the matter is that most of us find it difficult to change our behavior patterns from the ones that we have already established.

Our behavior patterns, or habits, can become so deeply ingrained, and the longer they have been part of our lives, the harder they can be to change. Most of us are aware that making poor food choices can lead to having too high of a calorie intake, raised cholesterol levels, and can be detrimental to our long-term health. However, there are many complex reasons why people might be motivated to choose unhealthy lifestyle habits. We also know that, based on scientific research, simply presenting someone with helpful information is not enough to actually result in real lifestyle change. Creating new and positive habits needs a mix of interventions. Trying to change everything we are doing within a very short time frame can feel very overwhelming. Moving very quickly to make big lifestyle changes also means that it is very difficult to maintain these new habits indefinitely. After all, that is the goal when trying to change your nutrition habits for good. The more overwhelmed we feel about making change, the more likely we will revert to our old habits. This is probably why we all have experienced our friends, family, and even coworkers telling us how they began a diet, had some positive results, but "fell off the wagon" again after a few weeks.

Many of the diets that we are familiar with do not even plan for long-term success. More often than not, they are set up to last for somewhere between thirty and sixty days. Then, after having worked through the program, there is little motivation to carry the big changes that we have made to our eating habits on with us into the future. No provision is made for assessing our progress or for setting new personal goals. The 'diet' does not help us with coping strategies for overcoming the hurdles which we will inevitably encounter. It seems very easy, then, to return to the comfort of those old, unhealthy habits which had been part of our lives for so long.

Chapter 1:

Change Your Nutrition,

Change Your Life!

However, there are ways that we can implement changes in our lives and establish them as positive habits. A drastic, all-encompassing change at the start of your better lifestyle journey is more likely to have limited results. This would be akin to deprivation, and as described already, we are less likely to achieve success if we feel that change is overwhelming. Based on some of the studies and the research that has been done on the most effective ways to make long-term changes to our diet, there are some simple steps we can take to change our nutrition habits for good.

Being well-informed about the foods that we should be eating is vital. We first should learn about the nutrient-dense, low calorie foods that our bodies need. We also need to be informed about proper hydration and how much water intake we should be getting to be fully hydrated. But just 'knowing' about the correct foods and the correct amount of food and water we should have on a daily basis is not enough. Slow, consistent change is the best way to achieve long-term change. Making small food substitutions and initially not cutting out all of the foods that were part of our old habits is key. We are less likely to crave sugar, unhealthy fats, and carbohydrates if we give ourselves enough time to adjust to this new way of eating. Slowly incorporating more of the fuel that we need: nutritious, high fiber, high protein, low calorie, vitamin, mineral-rich foods, and proper hydration at a gradual, methodical pace allows us time to get used to these changes.

While on our path to better health, we also need to take a self-monitoring approach. Recording our behavior, such as writing a food diary and assessing and taking stock of our progress, is important. Being able to set realistic, achievable goals for ourselves can help us move from step to step on this road to success. Learning to be proactive about problem-solving and finding coping strategies for the times when we "hit a wall" or begin to find things difficult is also something that can really help to make the changes we are thinking about permanent habits.

Part of the reason that breaking unhealthy habits can be so difficult is that we are creatures of habit. Our bodies naturally take on a rhythm or schedule. If you are unhappy with the way your diet is affecting your life and health, it is probably because you are already in a very comfortable rhythm and schedule that is not benefiting you. Evidence suggests that good time management techniques, planning ahead how you will fit your new shopping and meal preparation into your daily routine, can really help you to maintain this new lifestyle.

Chapter 2:

Step 1- Making Healthier

Food Choices

Most diets set us up for failure because most of them require us to make drastic dietary changes overnight. In this chapter, we will endeavor to get to the heart of how to finally make the changes you have been wanting and hoping to work toward. This approach is a pretty straightforward and simple one. However, please remember to talk with your doctor before making any changes to your nutrition and stay away from any foods you may be allergic.

Fruit

It is recommended that adults get between 1½-2 cups of fruit every day. Individuals who are more physically active may need more. (Fruits, 2020)

Fruit juices and dried fruit often have quite a bit of added sugar, so be on the lookout for that and focus more on whole fruits. Whole fruits are best for us. Try your best to mix it up and get a wide variety:

- Blackberries

- Blueberries

- Strawberries

- Bananas

- Grapefruit

- Pineapple

- Apples

- Cherries

- Olives

- Cranberries

This list is comprised of some of the healthiest fruits out there, all full of vitamins, minerals, and fiber. (Davidson, 2021)

Vegetables

It is recommended that adults get between 2½-3 cups daily. Again, those that are more physically active may need more. (Vegetables, 2020)

- Carrots

- Brussels Sprouts

- Spinach

- Broccoli

- Kale

- Garlic

- Green Peas

- Ginger

- Asparagus

- Swiss Chard

- Sweet Potatoes

- Collard Greens

This list is comprised of some of the healthiest vegetables out there! (Raman, 2021) In the same way, as with the fruit, try to mix it up and get a wide variety. Eating vegetables of all different colors means you are working toward getting the many different vitamins and minerals that we need, and we need a wide variety of those too.

Grains

It is recommended that adults get 3-8 ounce equivalents each day. Individuals engaging in more physical activity may require more. (Grains, 2020) Whole grains are the aim here.

- Whole Oats

- Millet

- Whole Wheat

- Whole Grain Rye

- Buckwheat

- Brown Rice

- Quinoa

- Whole Grain and Whole Wheat Pastas

This list is comprised of some of the healthiest grains out there. (Raman, 2021)

These fruits, vegetables, and grains are all high in fiber. The fiber found in these foods is essential to controlling blood sugar. Getting all these foods in these amounts will slow the absorption of sugar into the bloodstream, keeping your blood sugar in a healthy range and stop it from spiking. (Harvard Health Publishing, 2017) Why is this important? Put simply, when our blood sugar levels spike, especially for prolonged periods of time, our bodies are more likely to store body fat. That's one reason why our body fat can increase so much, and we can become overweight. (Burns, 2021) Many of us get too much processed sugar, too little fiber, too little water, too much caffeine, and too little exercise. This combination can lead to unwanted health concerns.

Proteins

For adults, it is recommended to get 5-6½ ounce equivalents per day. It is also best to get protein from a variety of sources, preferably lean, low-fat options. (Protein, 2020)

- Tuna

- Lean Beef

- Eggs

- Lentils

- Pumpkin Seeds

- Almonds

- Chicken Breast

- Turkey Breast

- Fish

- Oats

- Greek Yogurt

This list contains some of the most nutritious proteins out there. (Gunnars, 2021)

For more information about all these foods, go to myplate.gov. Also, consult with your physician or nutritionists before changing your diet.

Chapter 3:

Step 2 - Record What You

Are Eating

For at least one week, record everything you eat. Then, compare that to the recommendations in this guide. See what you do well with and what needs improvement. During this step, don't try to improve your diet at all. This is simply to give yourself an honest look at how you are currently fueling your body.

Snacking

When you begin recording your food intake, you may be surprised at the amount of incidental food (snacks) that you are eating every day. Snacking is not automatically bad; what is important is what we are snacking on and how much we are eating. If you find that you are snacking a lot, you may decide to snack less and less over time with a clear, specific plan to move forward. Otherwise, you may decide to start slowly changing the foods you are snacking on as well as the amount per serving/per day. You may also decide to try a combination of these, such as changing what you are snacking on first and then removing snacking altogether at a later point. It really is all about what you are comfortable changing and will stick to long-term. If you are snacking on the foods mentioned in this guide and aren't getting more than the daily recommended amount per category, then snacking can be perfectly fine.

Water

One of the most important considerations when changing to better eating habits is water. Being properly hydrated all day, every day, is vital. The cells in our body that work to allow every bodily function to happen need to be properly hydrated so that they can operate at their optimum. In other words, if you are dehydrated, your skin gets drier and can become flakey. Your mouth gets dry, and it can be harder to swallow. If you are not properly hydrated, it is harder to digest food as well. Your heart has a harder time pumping blood because blood gets thicker the less hydrated it is. Your circulation can become worse. Your blood vessels can constrict more. You may experience more headaches. The body's ability to deliver nutrients to different parts that may need repair becomes hampered.

Your muscles can start to cramp. Your energy levels can drop, causing fatigue.

The human body NEEDS water, and we are constantly using water and losing water that needs to be replaced often. The bottom line is that water is good, and we need it! So how much do we need? A good rule of thumb is to take your body weight in pounds and divide this by two. (Stone, 2019) The number that you get is how many ounces you need per day to stay properly hydrated. When you are recording your diet before you begin making changes, also remember to think about how much water you are drinking. This may be one of the changes that you will need to make in order to achieve the healthy lifestyle that you are hoping for in life. Again, before you change anything about your nutrition, please consult your physician to be sure that it is right for you.

Chapter 4:

Step 3 - Plan Your Steps to

Success

Properly planning the changes that you intend to make is another important key to success. First, pick just one or two things you want to improve. Perhaps you would like to start with getting more water and vegetables. Or maybe you would like to begin by getting more grains and fruits. Either way, it is important to make only slight changes every month CONSISTENTLY, until eventually, you are getting everything in the recommended amounts every day. Over time, you will get used to eating in this way. You will find that you will not even have to think twice about it, as your new eating behaviors will become new healthy habits.

Consistent Progress

Creating a concrete plan, including only one or two changes at a time that is achievable, and setting a clear time limit for yourself to reach your goals and set new ones is a very positive start on your journey to a healthier lifestyle. As mentioned already, being consistent with your new eating behaviors and sticking to your plans are most important. Without consistency, we really would find it difficult to accomplish anything. Learning to play an instrument, becoming an architect, learning a new language, improving strength and endurance, working toward a promotion require consistent effort and practice. To achieve any of these things requires that our behavior be aligned with achieving the goal at hand, and we need to engage in our new goal-oriented behaviors (you guessed it) CONSISTENTLY. Without consistency, we will fail to reach the goal.

Think about improving your nutrition in the same way as you would at getting better at the piano. In order to become a competent pianist, you have to practice a couple of times a week or more. Eventually, you play more and more often as you improve a little at a time. Changing our eating behaviors is the same. Slowly and steadily, chop away at bad behaviors while slowly and steadily adding better ones. Think of something in your life that you have accomplished over time that you were not able to master immediately. Something that took a consistent amount of practice over months, or even years! Think about how you approached achieving this goal and how you were able to stick with it. You most likely worked at it a little every day or a few times a week and slowly made progress until you hit your target. Let's apply this same approach to your nutrition habits!

Chapter 5:

Step 4 - Scheduling

Grab a calendar and start scheduling! Use the calendar and reminder applications on your phone, or use an actual paper calendar and begin to schedule in the same 1-3 days per week for the next four weeks to implement your plan. Think positively! Once you get going and are eating better than you were before you started, then you are on the right track. If you feel stuck, ask yourself why you feel that way. Also, remind yourself that you have made progress and are eating better now than you were. It's ok to hit a wall. Life likes to throw us curveballs. Even the smallest change is good as long as it is an improvement to what you are currently doing. For example, one extra cup of water one day a week or an extra serving of broccoli on Thursdays. Even these small changes can be considered progress.

Start with targets that are small and feel that they can be made permanent. An example of an unrealistic permanent change is going from drinking 1-2 cups of water per day now to, starting tomorrow, drinking 12 cups of water per day and expecting to stick to that for the rest of your life. I'm sure most of us remember the tale of the tortoise and the hare. The tortoise had it right. SLOW and STEADY wins this race, in health.

Chapter 6:

Step 5 - Assessing Your

Progress

Self-monitoring and creating your own personalized plan are where things start to come together. The more specific and realistic you can be, the more likely it is that you will succeed and adhere to your plan indefinitely. Here is an example: let's say I decide I need to get more water and more vegetables based on the daily recommendations. After recording what I am actually eating, I can see that I am only getting, on average, one cup of vegetables per day. I should be getting three cups per day. In the past, I have tried to drastically increase my vegetable intake every day and gave up after two weeks because it was overwhelming. This is one of the important things to remember: AVOID FEELING OVERWHELMED!

This is the reason we quit doing the things that will get us where we want to be. So instead of trying to get three cups every day, schedule yourself to get 2-2½ cups 1-3 days per week on the same days at the same meals (breakfast, lunch, or dinner). Also, pinpoint what those vegetables will be for the next four weeks. The same principle applies to water intake. Now you have a very specific game plan to follow. It is only for 1-3 days per week (much easier to accomplish and stick to long-term) instead of trying to do it every day (overwhelming and therefore short-lived). Now, you can get into a rhythm and allow your body to get used to the changes.

Your rate of progress will depend on your adherence and your acceptance of the nutritional behavior changes. Your adherence will depend on how comfortable and easy the changes make you feel. The way you know whether you can be more aggressive or if you need to slow down is how easy the four-week blocks are. If you start off with two days per week where you increase your vegetable intake from 1 to 2-2 ½ cups on those days, and that change feels easy and manageable to the point where you think you could do that for the rest of your life, then you can congratulate yourself. You are succeeding!

The best diet you can ever go on is one that is better than what you are doing now, as well as one you can do forever. Now, if you can do this consistently for four weeks, then you can increase the number of days per week to get the extra cups of vegetables by 1-2 days. Try that for another four weeks, and so on. Keep repeating this process until you reach seven days a week and feel comfortable with the nutrition behavior changes you have made. If you begin to feel overwhelmed, you can slow down again until you feel comfortable. The length of time it takes to adapt varies from person to person.

Once you have mastered this and you feel that you can easily maintain that new behavior, then move on to the next goal, whether that is to increase your water intake or add more fruits, grains, or proteins to your diet. The timeline can vary depending on your current nutrition behaviors relative to your nutrition goals and could take anywhere from two months to 24+ months. We are not trying to change everything about our nutrition all at once (think of how many times trying this has led to failure for you or someone you know). Instead, we are going for slow and CONSISTENT change by tackling only one or two categories at a time. That consistency will lead to permanent behavior changes that will change your life!

Chapter 7:

What Motivates Us?

Most of us who feel that we need to change our nutritional habits are already somewhat aware that many of the food choices we are making are not the most healthy. We are exposed to facts every day in the media and on social media about healthy diets and healthy lifestyles. We can easily access the information we need to help us to choose foods with better nutritional value. Why, then, is it so difficult for us to make these changes and adopt better habits that we can sustain and enable us to lead healthier lives?

There are many different theories about motivation and what drives us to behave in particular ways. There is very rarely a simple, clear-cut reason why people eat and drink things that they know are not good for them. One suggestion might be that for some people who have already tried 'dieting,' the amount of work they had to do to stay on a diet seemed too difficult, and the results were not rewarding enough. We are always looking for the path of least resistance. If the effort we have to expend to make the change we want is harder than what we are already doing, we resist. The more overwhelming, different, and drastic the changes, the harder it is for us to make these changes into new habits that we want to become part of our lifestyle. Eventually, for most, the easy thing to do is to fall back into our old ways.

Another reason why it might be difficult for us to maintain a healthy lifestyle is that we have low expectations of ourselves or of how much of a positive impact the changes we are thinking about making will have on our lives. Sometimes, this might result from a lack of self-confidence; we feel that we will never be able to achieve the outcome that we are hoping to see. If we have an underlying feeling that we will never be able to achieve our goals, it is much more difficult to find the motivation to begin working toward them. Also, a lack of information about what we need to do to change our unhealthy lifestyles, or even misinformation, can instill in us a fear of embarrassment. We worry that we will not know how to overcome the inevitable barriers that we will find in our way, and we never set out on the journey.

A third reason why changing to healthier eating habits might be difficult is that, and it has to be acknowledged, a lot of the foods we eat that are of little nutritional value taste good. They give us an immediate dopamine hit that we enjoy and get pleasure. When we eat foods with higher sugar content, for example, they release chemicals that fuel our body's natural 'reward' system, and they make us feel good for a short period of time. With processed foods and sugary foods being so easily accessible and affordable for most of us, it is only natural that many people will find themselves being tempted into including a lot of these in their diet. Unfortunately, the more sugar we eat, the more we can often find ourselves craving sugar, and this can become almost addictive. A sudden change of diet where we remove all sugary foods can also cause resistance within us. We can find this difficult to maintain, and a similar pattern emerges. We cave in, give in, and give up. It all seems just too hard. The message here is to give yourself small, measurable, achievable targets, take the time you need to self-monitor and assess your progress and be as consistent with your changes as you can be.

Don't forget to consult with your physician before making any lifestyle, exercise, or nutrition changes. Following these simple steps can help you implement changes to your nutrition that will change your life; safety is important!

Conclusion

Any major changes that we make in our lives can be difficult. Whether that is changing jobs, moving house, ending a relationship, or planning a family- all of these things can seem overwhelming at the outset. Embarking upon a lifestyle overhaul can seem just as overwhelming! As stated in the previous chapter, most of us who are thinking about changing to a healthier lifestyle are already aware that the choices we are making now are not the best ones for us. We perhaps know that we are not as active as we should be, that we are eating too many highly processed and sugary foods, or that we do not include enough nutritious fruits and vegetables in our diet. However, the thought of changing all of these things within a thirty or sixty-day time frame can seem impossible, and it may be difficult to muster up the motivation to get started.

In order to avoid falling off the wagon or "abandoning ship" early on in the process of trying to make nutritional changes or, worse still, being too overwhelmed to even know where to begin, we need to remember that creating better eating habits takes time. As previously mentioned, just like learning an instrument or any other new skill for the first time, changing the way that you eat and fuel your body requires some consistent effort and is not going to happen overnight!

The message here is that we need to create smaller, more manageable goals for ourselves so that the 'finish line' does not always seem so far away! Choosing only one or two changes to make at a time is key. In this way, we do not feel like we are depriving ourselves of anything, and we are more likely to be able to consistently stick to the healthier lifestyle that we are wanting. Planning a realistic time frame within which to implement those changes is also crucial. If you are able to maintain one or two healthier changes for a four-week period, it is then very realistic to think that you could then re-assess and re-set your targets and make another one or two positive changes in the next four weeks. Creating 'SMART' lifestyle goals (small, measurable, attainable, realistic, and time-based) enables us to make 'smart' changes to our nutrition that we are more likely to be able to keep for life! After all, that is the ultimate goal!

References

Behaviour Change Models and Strategies: (EUFIC). (2014). Eufic.org. https://www.eufic.org/en/healthy-living/article/motivating-behaviour-change

Burns, E. (2021). *How Elevated Blood Sugar Causes Weight Gain (and What to Do About It).* Nutracraft. https://www.nutracraft.com/blogs/weight-loss/how-elevated-blood-sugar-causes-weight-gain-and-what-to-do-about-it

Cristol, H. (2019, June 19). *What Is Dopamine?* WebMD; WebMD. https://www.webmd.com/mental-health/what-is-dopamine

Davidson, K. (2021, May 10). *20 Tasty Fruits with Health Benefits.* Healthline. https://www.healthline.com/nutrition/healthy-fruit#TOC_TITLE_HDR_10

Fruits | MyPlate. (2020). Www.myplate.gov. https://www.myplate.gov/eat-healthy/fruits

Gunnars, K. (2020, March 3). *20 Delicious High Protein Foods to Eat.* Healthline. https://www.healthline.com/nutrition/20-

delicious-high-protein-
foods#TOC_TITLE_HDR_2

Hardcastle, S. J., Hancox, J., Hattar, A., Maxwell-Smith, C., Thøgersen-Ntoumani, C., & Hagger, M. S. (2015). *Motivating the unmotivated: how can health behavior be changed in those unwilling to change?* Frontiers in Psychology, 6(6:835). https://doi.org/10.3389/fpsyg.2015.00835

Harvard Health Publishing. (2017, May). *The sweet danger of sugar - Harvard Health.* Harvard Health; Harvard Health. https://www.health.harvard.edu/heart-health/the-sweet-danger-of-sugar

Link, R. (2017, May 14). *The 14 Healthiest Vegetables on Earth.* Healthline. https://www.healthline.com/nutrition/14-healthiest-vegetables-on-earth#TOC_TITLE_HDR_16

Protein Foods | MyPlate. (2020). Www.myplate.gov. https://www.myplate.gov/eat-healthy/protein-foods

Raman, R. (2018, July 14). *14 Healthy Whole-Grain Foods (Including Gluten-Free Options).* Healthline. https://www.healthline.com/nutrition/whole-grain-foods

Grains | MyPlate. (2020). Www.myplate.gov. https://www.myplate.gov/eat-healthy/grains

Stone, J. (2019). *How to calculate how much water you should drink | University of Missouri System.* Www.umsystem.edu. https://www.umsystem.edu/totalrewards/welln ess/how-to-calculate-how-much-water-you-should-drink/

Vegetables | MyPlate. (2020). Www.myplate.gov. https://www.myplate.gov/eat-healthy/vegetables

Why food deprivation doesn't work. (2017, September 14). Well+Good. https://www.wellandgood.com/food-deprivation-healthy-eating-weight-watchers/

Printed in Great Britain
by Amazon

42625367R00030